Squirt Stories

Squirt Stories

Tales of Real Life Squirters

R. LEIGH

This book is dedicated to all the brave women who stepped up to share intimate details of themselves, who in turn will encourage another woman to embrace her sexuality, let go, and unleash her flood.

Thank you to the wonderful ladies located from all parts of the world who were willing to share their stories. Although some of them were hesitant, they were brave enough to share such intimate parts of themselves. Sexuality is a difficult area for many women to embrace, but through hearing others' stories, women are sometimes able to realize they are no different than anyone else and we all have desires which are not so unusual, and it's perfectly acceptable to enjoy sex.

Contents

Other Books by Author

Squirting: It's Easier Than You Think: A Holistic Guide to Female Pleasure, available on Amazon.com and BarnesandNoble.com.

COWARD: Becoming Courageous: The Struggle to Leave an Abusive Relationship and Learn to Like Yourself Again, available on Amazon.com.

Also check out Squirt School. More information can be found on www.AuthorRLeigh.com.

Why I Wrote This Book

Before I wrote *Squirting: It's Easier Than You Think: A Holistic Guide to Female Ejaculation*, it was primarily men who wanted to talk to me about squirting. Part of me began to question if there were other squirters like me, even though I knew there were. But writing the book opened up the conversation, and women began to tell me their stories. Many of these stories mimicked my own, but every woman was distinctly different in how they first started squirting, what it's like for them, and even how they feel about being a squirter. Although I would say every woman I encountered felt it is an enjoyable experience.

Through this book I want to share with you the stories of some real life squirters. Not porn stars, but your next door neighbor, the mom down the street, the person you cross in the grocery store. Women who are enjoying this phenomenon in the privacy of their bedrooms.

I think, like myself (especially initially), some women question this ability, their comfortableness with it, if it's acceptable, etc. I think through reading these stories you'll understand everyday women just like you experience female ejaculation.

1

Squirting: The New Orgasm?

As sexuality evolves, squirting could become the "new orgasm." At one time clitoral orgasms were the main orgasm. Then the g-spot orgasm became the holy grail of orgasms. The squirting orgasm is the one more and more people are talking about, and with some help and knowledge, more and more women will have the ability to achieve them, and the end goal could become squirting, even if the fluid is in smaller quantities than the large amounts some women project (remember porn sensualizes everything, and some women's ejaculate is in much smaller quantities). Because for a man, the act seems unfinished if he does not ejaculate. So more and more women may begin to feel their orgasm is only complete if they also ejaculate.

While squirting has clearly been around for a long time, it's just now becoming more mainstream.

Check out this timeline of the history of squirting:

- Scholars began describing female ejaculation about 2,000 years ago.

- Tantric sex practitioners called it Amrita, the nectar of the goddess.

- Fourth century Chinese Taoist texts referred to the female prostate (i.e. the g-spot) as a moon flower that gushes large amounts of nectar. Chinese poetry even talks about milk fruit (the G-spot) and how a man can stimulate this area with his finger or penis tip to bring forth female honey.

- The Kamasutra, which dates to 200-400 A.D., speaks of female semen falling continually.

- The Greek philosopher Aristotle spoke of female ejaculation, pointing out it exceeds the quantity of what a man ejaculates.

- In the 17th century, the Dutch physician Reinier De Graaf explained how the periurethral glands were the female version of the male prostate and the source of female ejaculatory fluid. This was considered the first truly scientific account of female ejaculation.

- In 1952 the German physician Ernest Gräfenberg was credited with "discovering" an erotic zone on the anterior wall of the vagina running along the course of the urethra. This is what we now know is the g-spot. Gräfenberg observed masturbating women expelling fluids from their urethra with orgasm "in gushes." Since this never occurred at the beginning of sexual stimulation, but rather only at the time of orgasm, the physician concluded that its purpose was more for pleasure than for lubrication. Gräfenberg wrote that the fluid was examined and it had no urinary character. He said the fluid expelled during female orgasm is not urine, but instead secretions of the intraurethral glands.

- The discussion began again in 1980 when a groundbreaking book called The G-*spot* was released. The G-*Spot* was the first book to prove the existence and define the location of the Gräfenberg spot, or the G-spot, as a patch of erectile tissue.

In past years squirting was largely absent from porn. In 2014, Pornhub reported the term "squirt" as the seventh most searched term worldwide. In some areas of the world it ranks even higher; in the UK it's the fourth most popular search term, and not surprisingly at least half of my book sales come from the UK. It's a popular searched term in porn, men love to experience it, and while not all women are experiencing it, many have experienced it by accident (that's the most common way a woman discovers she can squirt). Women search on the term almost twice as much as men, proving women are interested in experiencing a squirting orgasm, or have had one and weren't aware of what it was when it happened. While our focus has been on clitoral or g-spot orgasms, now squirting is more widely discussed. It is my belief that in the next 10 or so years, most women, and men, will recognize squirting as a normal orgasm.

2

Seeking Squirters

When I put out the call looking for squirters (via my website and mentions on several radio interviews) one of the first emails I received was from a woman excited that there "is a larger community of squirters." Most "normal," everyday women don't openly talk about female ejaculation, I think leaving most to believe they are maybe the only one doing it, or at least part of a small club. Most squirters seem to feel they are a unique anomaly when they admit to a man (or woman) they can squirt. Yet it's also exciting when a man (or woman) is intrigued and excited because he's (she's) "never been with a squirter," a comment I've heard almost every time I've had a new partner. But along with the intrigue and excitement comes some shame and embarrassment as women often wonder if it's normal, if it's acceptable, or even if their partner truly enjoys it.

The initial response to my call for squirters was overwhelming, yet I received much fewer submissions in return. Initially, I took it personally. I thought something in my approach was turning people off. Was it something I said? A question I asked? Did I ask too many questions? So I decided to start asking why my respondents weren't following through in writing their stories. I'm glad I did for my own peace of mind, but I was disheartened by what I heard in response because their response is exactly why I wrote not only this book, but my first book about squirting as well. The women who were contacting me felt sexually mature and adventurous, but when it came to discussing sexuality in such detail it made them uncomfortable. There was still a level of shame. It was too difficult to talk about their sexuality in such great detail. While they felt sexually open, writing a narrative was too uncomfortable, too vulnerable. Most of them (like me) had experienced past sexual trauma or had been taught shame about the subject. I also consider myself fairly comfortable with my sexuality, but yet I still experience a level of shame. There is embarrassment in writing both of my books. It's not something I would ever want my family, and even some of my friends to read, but I wrote them because I felt I was supposed to, and I believe following where you are led will only lead you to the right places.

So many of my life experiences make me feel as though I was brought to this point. From my rape to molestation at the hands of more than one adult, as well as growing up in an environment where sexuality was barely discussed. I feel as though I was prepared to go on a journey to discover healthy sexuality, and share it with others. So much of the sex in our society, particularly in the United States, is shame-based, or so many bad things happen to people whether it's rape, molestation, STD's, etc. But I don't believe sex is supposed to be bad. I don't believe it's supposed to be shameful. And if we've had bad sexual experiences, such as rape, I don't believe we are supposed to remain locked in that experience, to never again experience a fulfilling, healthy sex life.

I shared much of my own story about my squirting experiences in my first book *Squirting: It's Easier Than You Think*. Much of it was shared with reservation, and I still doubt if I should have shared such a private part of my life. Yet, why I did has much more to do with my belief that it could help someone. When I had my first squirting experience I was uninformed and uneducated. Where do normal, everyday people learn about such things? Not within sexual education. Not from our parents. Porn is probably where most people learn about it. And if you've read my first book or listened to any of the multiple interviews I've done, you'll know I wasn't a porn watcher, nor do I believe porn is an effective form of sex education. Much of it is based around theatrics and to shock. Much of it is not real.

3

Sexual Repression

Sexual repression: a state in which a person is prevented from expressing his or her sexuality. Sexual repression is often associated with feelings of guilt or shame being associated with sexual impulses. What constitutes sexual repression is subjective and can vary greatly between cultures and moral systems. Many religions have been accused of fostering sexual repression. ~Wikipedia

We still have double standards for men and women. A woman's sexuality is still largely repressed. If a man has sex with many women he is a player or even admired, and his behavior is socially acceptable. Yet, if a woman has sex with more than a few men, and even sometimes if she is sexually adventurous, she is considered a whore or a slut, the kind of woman you have fun with, but don't marry. Even other women will attribute such characteristics to her.

In all actuality a woman can be conservative and monogamous and enjoy sex, and at the same time have great sexual desires. Some women may prefer to be less monogamous, and may desire more partners.

Female genital mutilation is still the norm in certain parts of the world, yet interestingly enough, women are multi-orgasmic and are the only sex which possess the only body part (the clitoris) whose sole purpose is pleasure. Talk about repression!

We want to believe we are enlightened about sex, but in society as a whole, we still are not.

What does sexual repression have to do with squirting? The ability to squirt is directly tied to the ability for a woman to let go, to be animalistic, to feel comfortable getting dirty, to let go of mental blocks, to let go of any ideas around sexual repression. She has to have the mindset that pleasure is acceptable. Squirting (or the lack of being able to) is directly tied to this concept of sexual repression among women and their inability to embrace and enjoy their sexuality in spite of outside societal opinions and judgments.

4

———

A Discussion about Gender Equality (or Gender Inequality)

Gender inequality: unequal treatment or perceptions of individuals based on their gender. It arises from differences in socially constructed gender roles as well as biologically through chromosomes, brain structure, and hormonal differences. ~Wikipedia

In 2015, gender equality is a hot topic, and there is a shift underway. Our children, and our children's children will see a change in how women are valued, no doubt about it. And gender equality is relevant in every area, even sexuality.

The Gender Equality Division of the Department of Justice and Equality in Ireland says, "Gender equality is achieved when women and men enjoy the same rights and opportunities across all sectors of society, including economic participation and decision-making, and when the different behaviours, aspirations, and needs of women and men are equally valued and favoured."

Pay attention to that last part, "the behaviours and needs of women and men are equally valued." While gender equality most often refers to income, or the socioeconomic status of women, it can refer to sexuality as well, and does. Sexuality is a daily part of who we are and what we do. We are born sexual beings.

While sexual repression and gender inequality are two separate terms, they are related.

Gender stereotypes are difficult to break, and whether we like to admit it or not, we are all prone to engaging in stereotyping at one time or another.

5

Introduction to the Stories

What's still discouraging to me is while many women contacted me, few actually stepped up and followed through to share their stories. Because of the intimacy of the subject, even though they would remain anonymous, as I've mentioned, few women seemed truly comfortable discussing the subject in much detail. Yet, openly talking about the subject is how we learn and form an understanding of any subject.

One of the participants in this book (who shall rename nameless) backed out of the project initially, saying she wanted to participate, but yet she just couldn't.

When I asked her way she didn't feel she could participate, this was her response: "You know, I'm not entirely sure. I'm certainly not a prude. I am very uninhibited sexually, I love it as part of a relationship or on its own. The consensus is I'm really good at it. But I just can't talk about it. I was raised by a woman who tolerated sex because she knew it was an important part of marriage. We grew up knowing sex was bad. We knew this because it was NEVER talked about. But I still can't really talk about it. I guess it's that childhood of denial, that little bit I can't get rid of."

I'm glad she decided to share her story after we talked further.

To give you some insight here are the questions I asked these willing participants to answer in writing their narratives about their experience.

- How long have you been squirting?

- When did it first happen? How old were you? Explain the scenario in which it happened?

- Where you expecting it?

- Did you know what it was? What was your knowledge of squirting?

- How did you feel about it at the time?

- Was it pleasurable?

- Did you seek to make it happen again?

- Have your partners been happy with the experience?
  Have you ever had any partners who weren't or who were grossed out by the experience?

- How do you address it with a new partner? If a partner is grossed out by it, how do you handle it?

- How do you handle the mess?

- What do you do in order to squirt? What tricks have you learned? Are there certain toys you use?

- Is it easier to squirt via masturbation or with a partner?

- Is there anything specific your partner does which allows you to squirt? Has your ability to squirt (and what works) varied with different partners?

- Do you squirt every time you have sex, or every time you masturbate?

- How long does it take you to squirt?

- How has squirting changed over the years, as you've become more experienced with it?

- Have you ever experienced problems with having any type of orgasm, receiving pleasure during sex, etc.? Many women struggle with staying in their head, or worrying about how they look, taste, etc. This affects all types of orgasms.

- Have you had any strange experiences occur because of or when you were having a squirting orgasm?

- What is your knowledge of squirting? What do you think

the fluid is made up of? Why does it happen? Have you researched much about it (some squirters seem to since they are taken by surprise when it happens)?

• Do you think every woman has the ability to squirt? If not, why do you think some women can't?

These stories are unedited, except for spelling errors or to address any major clarity issues. I wanted these remarkable women's voices to be heard. This means some of the writing may be a bit messy, but beautiful. A beautiful mess…I'd describe squirting the same way.

So with that introduction I leave you with these stories.

6

CASSIE

27 years old, Mother of 1, Student, cohabitating with her boyfriend, United States

I've been squirting since I met my most recent boyfriend....about 5 months.

It happened at age 27, after a few times of being intimate with my current boyfriend. We were very connected emotionally, exposed ourselves emotionally very early, and I think that had a lot to do with it. I was very comfortable in my own skin and my own body this time that we made love. I was on top and he is a very sturdy 7 inches. I believe this is the first time I experienced a cervical orgasm. He penetrated (I believe), briefly my cervix, and I squirted several times in about a 10 minute period.

I wasn't expecting it. Not in the slightest. Even with my

husband, or other previous lovers, I did not experience anything close to an orgasm during intercourse.

I didn't know what it was. I literally asked my boyfriend "what did you just do?" It seems he was actually on a mission, and is a very educated man, in regards to the needs and anatomy of women. BIG DEAL. Makes a world of difference. He wanted to make me squirt. I thought it was a myth.

After the first time I never wanted to have sex the old way again.

I can't get enough. I never used to initiate sex. My ex-husband was a user. He'd land me for 5 minutes, get his willies off and then fall asleep. I was left to my own devices after that, if I didn't feel violated, that is.

I DEFINITELY sought to make it happen again after the first time.

My boyfriend, the only partner I have right now, and the only person who has helped me squirt, loves when it happens. He feels rewarded for his hard work, which it isn't so hard to do anymore. We know a rhythm. I know what we are looking for, and so does he. I always get off first, and me getting off almost always makes him get off. Plus, lubrication is key anyways, so making me squirt just makes sense!!

We handle the mess by using a towel and then we take a shower.

Top is best. Touching the cervix makes a big difference. Can't do it with just anyone, I don't think, because you have to feel comfortable. Sex is in the woman's mind. If I'm not into it, I don't even try. I say no, and I never hear any grief. (This is the way it should be.)

I can only squirt with a partner. I cant make myself squirt. I can sure make myself get off, but it's not near as fun.

With my current partner, I squirt every time we have sex. I never squirt during masturbation.

It doesn't take me long to squirt, and sometimes I squirt multiple times.

Only have a couple of months under my belt, but it has gotten easier to squirt.

I don't have a clue [about squirting, what the fluid is, etc.]. I just go with it. Its better than any other sex I've ever known.

I think every woman has the ability to squirt, just has to be with the right guy, she needs to get out of her head. The guy has to be concerned with her pleasure. And size does matter, to me at least.

7

FIONA

48 years old, straight, in a relationship but currently live separately, professional career, no kids and never been married, United States.

I began to notice I was squirting around the age of 24 or 25. I'd been sexually active since I was 17 so it was a number of years, 8-9 years before I really discovered this talent!

When it first happened I must have been squirting with my then boyfriend, and not really understood that it was happening. I felt very much in love with my boyfriend and probably had the most enjoyable sex life with him than I'd really ever had before. However, it was when I was overseas and I in fact slept with a former boyfriend that I really began to understand this was not "normal." The fluid was spraying into the air and he was really surprised, as I was, to see this, and I had no idea what it was, other than extreme "cumming" and orgasm.

I wasn't expecting it at all. I assumed that I must have been extremely turned on and unusually sexually excited. Was it because I was in fact cheating on my boyfriend with a former boyfriend and it was a thrill? I wondered but in fact, it became the norm as opposed to the exception.

I was quite confused when it first happened, but not unhappy. I was excited by the idea that I could orgasm with such ease and voracity. It was very pleasurable. Once I understood how much effect a pronounced orgasm could have on my sexual partner, and on my sexual abilities, I was very keen to make it happen again, and again!

Pretty much every partner or sexual encounter I have had since then has been happy with the experience.

With new partners, I never address the issues of squirting in advance. I might say "this could get messy" which only creates a sense of intrigue. And they are always surprised and delighted! I have never experienced someone being grossed out. One sexual partner I dated briefly, told me a year later that the sex we had, and the way I came while sitting on his cock, was so exciting and so new, he masturbated to that thought for a year afterwards. Having said that, it could be that some men might freak out at the start and think I've urinated on them, however, it's never been raised as I feel they soon understand it's cum and they relax.

Oh the mess! Lots of towels and fresh sheets are needed. My mattress has a mattress protector. I have slept on towels many nights.

I wouldn't say I do anything specific to squirt. I simply relax and ensure I have full and complete enjoyment of the experience. At times I might engage in fantasy, but ideally I aim to be completely present throughout. Once that can be achieved then my partner will be the one to create the atmosphere and technique to allow me to squirt.

Mostly I squirt with a partner. There are times I squirt as I masturbate, but less so. I can squirt through clitoral stimulation, but for me to squirt fully I really need deep vaginal stimulation.

My current partner makes me squirt a great deal. Generally we find that clitoral stimulation to begin with, then he uses his fingers (two or three) on my g-spot, does a great job. However, one exciting development is that with him I am able to cum again and again during intercourse. Having said that, which I find exciting, there are times when he comments that it's so wet that he loses concentration, so that could be a downside!

I squirt most times when I have sex, unless I am very tired. I don't always squirt when I masturbate.

It generally takes only five to ten minutes for me to squirt.

My squirting has changed in the sense that it's easier to achieve than in the past, and seems to in fact travel further than ever. Recently my partner claims I squirted three feet.

I have always been fortunate with orgasms and not had a great deal of difficulty achieving them. I can orgasm multiple times in a sexual encounter. Some are more substantial than others, and they differ between clitoral and vaginal, so there is some variations in the orgasm.

I think flying cum is a very strange thing to see, but I don't believe I've had any other strange experiences. I find that after numerous orgasms I can feel dizzy and somewhat disoriented.

I have wondered a great deal about the content of the fluid. At times it smells somewhat like urine, but not that often, although it's not without smell. I believe there is not enough information out there about it at all. I recall once reading that it was part of a "super orgasm" which is when a woman has a deep connection between her mind and her genitals.

I don't believe that every women has the ability to squirt in the same way that not all women can orgasm, but it would be wonderful if all women could! Perhaps it's more about feeling confident within yourself and a more relaxed approach to sexuality. I have always felt very open in regards to sexuality and as such, every experience I have enjoyed and found great pleasure throughout my life.

8

JULIA

Age 57, happily married with 2 grown children, work in community health (nursing background), live in the south of England, essentially heterosexual (I say essentially, I have had some experience of sex with my own gender, but not for quite a few years now!).

I went through menopause 5 years ago, but that was not a happy experience, so I am now on Hormone Replacement Therapy which is the best invention since sliced bread as far as I am concerned!

Looking back, I think I have been someone who could ejaculate right from my teens, though back then I had absolutely no idea what was going on! As far as I was concerned, I was merely someone who got really very wet when aroused! To be honest, the concept of female ejaculation didn't arise until I was into my twenties, by then I had already had my first bad reaction to how wet I could get when a guy who was a few years older than me (I was 17 at the time) and who clearly had the manual skills to bring me to a climax (far more skilfully than the inexperienced lads I had been fooling around with up until then), promptly accused me of peeing all over the back seat of his precious Ford Cortina! I walked away from that encounter feeling rather deflated and embarrassed. I should point out that my ejaculations didn't "spurt" out (I dislike the word squirt as it now has the wrong connotations thanks to the adult film industry), they merely dribbled out. I suppose that I became a bit self-conscious when having sex following that, I was always aware that some guys might not find my wetness such a turn on. It wasn't until I was going through what I call my "all men are bastards" phase following a bitter break up with my then boyfriend that I found solace in the arms of another female who took me to places sexually that I didn't realize existed! It was during our first night together that she made me reach what was to be my first of several orgasms making me ejaculate in the process. This was a proper ejaculation…no dribbling out! The fluid spurted out quite unexpectedly as she was fingering me with her index finger while rubbing my clitoris with the ball of her thumb, I felt the orgasm welling up, but I was so wrapped up in the moment that I just let myself go. For a second or two I was mortified, I really thought that I had peed over her hand! Fortunately, she was already well versed in the mysteries of female ejaculation, she calmed me down and managed to convince me that what had just happened was indeed a rare and wonderful experience!

It's worth saying here that 6 months later I married the "bastard!" He, like the majority of male sexual partners I have had, was quite fascinated by my wetness, taking it as an affirmation of their sexual skills and not realizing that what I was experiencing was female ejaculation. Up until that fling with another female (I was 21) my ejaculations were more of a trickle rather than a squirt (or spurt as I prefer to call it). What it did do was frustrate me and confuse me, back in the mid/late 70s there was precious little information on that subject, in fact there was none! The Internet age was a long way off yet and the medical books I had access to simply didn't touch on that subject. My husband was a very fastidious person and soon grew fed up with the mess female ejaculations can cause, he always moaned about the size of the wet patch in bed which gradually started to affect the frequency of our sexual relations. That, as well as other little foibles, put a strain on the marriage and 3 years later we were getting a divorce! This was in 1981 and for a 9 month period I had no relationships whatsoever (I even contemplated trying my luck with women again!), I quit my job and spent some time with an aunt of mine who lived in the States to see if I could get my head straight. I got back to the UK in the autumn of 1982 and within 6 weeks I had met the man who is now my husband of 29 years! Right from the outset sex with him was fabulous, not only was he experienced with female ejaculation, he revelled in making me ejaculate! With him it was and still is a case of "put a couple of bath towels on the sheets" and making me cum over and again! I still can have up to 10 or more ejaculations with him in a session.

I've already mentioned that I have struggled to get any good information on female ejaculation over the years, up until the late 80s there was nothing out there, I wasn't even that convinced that female ejaculation really existed, but then things started to take shape, a very close friend showed me an article in one of the more controversial women's magazines (Cosmopolitan I think) on the subject of orgasms that touched on the topic of female ejaculation, albeit only fleetingly. It was a further 10 years before I was able to start really researching this fascinating topic thanks to the Internet! But by then I had already started to build a picture of the workings of my orgasms. I noticed that my ability to have orgasms that were accompanied by ejaculations changed with my menstrual cycle. Around mid cycle when I was ovulating and at my most horny I found that I would ejaculate more, but in the days leading up to my period my ejaculations would subside and for the first 3 or 4 days after my period finished my ejaculations would likewise be less copious. Another thing that became obvious was what we were doing would influence my ejaculations, for instance certain positions could enhance my ejaculation, any position that saw me with my knees drawn up to my chest seemed to make me "squirt" more, also cowgirl positions where I could control the depth of penetration so that the glans of my husband's penis was in contact with my Gspot while I stimulated my clitoris would produce spectacular ejaculations!

As for my theories, well….. Some are based on personal

experience and some on what I have been able to glean from various Internet resources. Firstly I am now certain that all women produce the fluid in question, we all have the same plumbing after all! It comes from the para-urethral gland, also known as the Skene's gland, which then drains into the urethra via ducts. Bearing in mind that its composition has been shown to be the same as male seminal fluid (sugars, proteins & minerals) one has to ask what its purpose is. One theory suggests that it irrigates the vagina thus providing sperm with a pH friendly environment in which to swim. Sounds plausible to me! So why is it that some women can "squirt" while others can't? I believe that it all depends on a couple of factors. Just as some people produce more saliva than others or some produce more sweat than others, some of us produce more of this fluid than others! It then starts to "back up" along the urethra, which is where the other factor comes in. Those of us with strong pelvic floor muscles experience stronger muscle contractions when we orgasm which force this surplus fluid out under pressure, making it spurt out. For the record, I estimate that the volume of fluid that I expel varies between 10mls and 20mls per ejaculation, certainly nothing like the gushing that sprays all over the place portrayed in adult movies!

I've already touched on the effect my menstrual cycle has on my ability to ejaculate, should mention that the menopause also had a profound effect. While I was perimenopausal my periods were inconsistent to say the least and my libido started to wane. That coincided with a disruption to my orgasms and consequently my ejaculations.

When the menopause proper hit me my vaginal secretions dried up and I stopped ejaculating completely. However, as I said earlier, starting on HRT completely reversed the effects of the menopause, my libido returned and with it my vaginal secretions, my orgasms and most interestingly my ejaculations! I also believe that levels of arousal have an effect on ejaculation. I know that on occasions that I am very aroused I reach my first orgasm and ejaculation more rapidly and usually go on to have more orgasms than usual.

Now there are some who will read this & will say "no, no, no.... women don't ejaculate, what they are experiencing is stress incontinence". Well, I'm afraid you are so mistaken! To start with, I always empty my bladder before sex or masturbation, secondly the fluid I ejaculate is clear and odorless (it does have a salty tang to it), whereas my pee is most certainly NOT odorless and is a fairly deep shade of yellow and as the wet patch on bed sheets dries to leave nothing more than a slight watermark round the edge we can definitely say that my ejaculate does not contain urine.

One more thing I should add is a qualification of the term "orgasm." I am fortunate enough to be multi-orgasmic, what I experience is a succession of peaks followed by a series of "valleys" where the peaks are the orgasms and are more often than not accompanied by an ejaculation. I can have any number of these (10 or more is common) and in the "valleys" (the gaps between my orgasms) which can last anything from 2 or 3 minutes to 20 or 30 seconds, I can happily tolerate continued genital stimulation. However, after a while I drop into what is a deeper "valley" which takes noticeably longer to climb out of and this is the sign that I am building up to what is my big climax, a much more intense orgasm that lasts longer, is more of an all over body sensation but most interestingly does not come with an ejaculation! After that my whole genital area becomes a no go area as it is far too sensitive to be touched.

9

ROCHELLE

ROCHELLE, 35, graphic designer, female, fondly known as Shell,
live beachside on the Sunshine Coast [Australia], bisexual and live
with my male partner plus our three poodles.

Coming out of an eight year and largely sexless
relationship in Sydney, my move to Brisbane opened my
mind, body and soul. Just shy of 30, I gave myself permission
to explore my sexuality, connecting with men, women and
myself.

In the right position and with the right partner (or simply
through self-touch) I have always been generous with the
amount of fluid that I release, but it wasn't until I began
dating my current partner and exploring my sexuality with a
female friend that I learned the art of female ejaculation.

My first experience began with a day of unexpected
flirtation.

Saturday's were typically a morning of creativity followed by lunch at the pub with my (out & proud) friend Stace, as the guy I was beginning to date worked on Saturdays. But this Saturday was pouring with rain, typical of the beginning of cyclone season in Queensland.

Around lunchtime, Stace popped up on Skype Chat with a little message "Can I be open and honest with you?" Already feeling aroused, when Stace followed with "What kind of panties do you wear?" it led into an afternoon of sexual chat, wine, short stories and masturbation. By the time we had finished, my left hand was covered with juices and my body in a state of bliss.

Later that evening Steve arrived for dinner, with the scent of sex still in the air it didn't take long for our bodies to meet. Lifting my skirt and holding me against the dining table, perhaps the sexual tension and need was too great, but as he rode against my g-spot I found my juices exploding across his body and onto the floor.

It was a sensation onto its own, one that caught us both by surprise and an experience that has been sort after (and achieved) many times since.

Thankfully the first time we were balanced over timber floors, so the juices were easy to mop up. The second time I had the privilege of cumming with Stace's face ready and waiting, carefully balanced at the edge of her bed with my legs wrapped around her head. Her quilt bore whatever was left. From there on a towel has always been on standby for when the juices flow.

In the past couple years I have learned that multiple

orgasms increase the flow of juices and sensitivity of the g-spot in the lead up to a squirting event. My favourite ways to induce a squirting episode are by spending an afternoon with my favourite toys ending with a solid finger/fist session, with multiple clitoral and anal orgasms, or with a hot and heavy session with Steve (my now partner) followed by his fingers bringing on the ultimate climax.

The beauty is in the difference of each of these situations.

When it is you and only you, I would class female ejaculation as a spiritual experience. Being one and balanced between mind, body and spirit. There are no time frames, just time out to explore your body.

Bringing on a squirting experience with another woman is incredibly intimate and delicious. Indulging in a body that is so similar to your own adds to the eroticism and sensualisation of the experience. A woman knows how to answer your needs instinctively, and her lips respond with instant need.

With a man it's red hot urgency and lust, followed by a need to fulfill your needs of satisfaction, delight and pleasure, with the knowledge that he drove you to that point of enlightenment.

Having taken the piss out of a number of porn films when trying to educate grown men that women have three holes not two, I was initially amazed at the thickness and the sweet almost honey smell of the ejaculation, rather than the water (piss) that you see in the porn films.

Our bodies are sacred temples, capable of many remarkable things but only if our mind, body and soul are aligned.

I would recommend to any woman to have one afternoon to herself. Allow her fingers to explore and view herself in the mirror. Enjoy a clitoral orgasm, anal orgasm and female ejaculation – then educate their partner on what they want and how they like it. Sex will never be the same again.

10

————

SUSAN

Middle-aged, multiple partners, United States

This is in two parts. The first is just so you know how I got to where I am. The second is about the squirting.

My mother was born in the 20s. Women back then endured sex, they did not enjoy it or participate much. I heard my mother tell someone that, while she did not approve of pre-marital sex, she was very much in favor of anything that allowed her daughters to enjoy sex because she knew how important it is to a marriage. That is not the message that was communicated to me all my life to that point (I was about 20). The message my sister and I got was that sex is bad and wrong. We knew this because it was NEVER so much as mentioned. That's a lot of very deep programming to try to get past.

To give you an idea, when I was 12, on a weekend day

when everyone else in the family was outside or at a friend's, my mother very somberly and quietly said, "Susan, there's something we need to talk about." And she took me into the back bathroom, closed – and locked – the door. My parents never even closed the bathroom door. Anyway, she got out the equipment, and began to explain menstruation to me. In a hushed voice and somber expression. What does this tell a girl! And most of the women I know who are contemporaries have a very similar experience. Whoopi Goldberg even has a routine about it. I not only had no sex drive, I hardly felt anything the first few times I had sex. Nothing turned me on.

As time passed, that changed, of course. But there is still always that voice in the background telling me this is wrong and I'm a slut. Do I know that's absurd? Of course, I do. But childhood teachings can be very difficult to overcome. Most of us are run by tapes so deep and so old that we don't even know they exist. In fairness, I must add here that part of this is because I was never a popular kid, I never had a lot of friends. So, I had no one to talk to about it. You know, no "street corner" education.

Fast-forward a few decades and the consensus is, I've gotten pretty darned good at it. But there is ALWAYS a little bit a fear around it. I am assertive in bed, but I am not aggressive. I know guys like to be directed at least a little bit because they desperately want to make us happy. But it's still difficult for me to do that. (I keep practicing, though.) So, onto the subject at hand…

I squirted once over 30 years ago. I didn't know what it was and it never happened again until recently. I was told at first that only very few women do that. One guy recently told every woman will squirt given the proper stimulation. I don't know if that's true.

About 5 years ago, I was with a guy who got me to do it almost every time. This was during the year of my life when I had a lot of lovers, I don't even know how many. Very few of them could do it. Every once in a while, but not often. And I can try to talk a guy through how to do it for me, but it rarely helps. I don't know if I'm not clear enough or they don't listen or what. I even asked one guy – who was very good at it – what to tell other guys to help them, but that didn't make much difference, either.

All the guys I've known find my squirting very sexy. I was in a position to see it myself once, and it is sexy. And they love making me squirt, it's a real "win" for them.

I only ever squirt from G-spot orgasms. That may be universal, I don't know. But it's a very different orgasm than clitoral ones. It's not as intense for me, but it just keeps going. I call it a rolling orgasm. You know how from licking or stroking, you get this huge buildup and then this big release, and then you're done for at least several minutes? Not with G-spot. There's a build, but I just keep going. I have never had to take a break, I'll go as long as the guy will. Which is usually a good while because it's such a win for them to get me so dripping wet. I mean, I will soak the sheets. I put a towel under myself if I'm going to have to sleep in those sheets soon. They are honestly too wet to sleep in.

References

Pornhub Insights: 2014 Year in Review, http://www.pornhub.com/insights/2014-year-in-review

Gender Equality in Ireland: What is Gender Equality?, http://www.genderequality.ie/en/GE/Pages/WhatisGE

About the Author

R. Leigh is the author of *Squirting: It's Easier Than You Think: A Holistic Guide to Female Pleasure* and the Instructor/Creator of Squirt School. Also the author of *COWARD: Becoming Courageous: The Struggle to Leave an Abusive Relationship and Learn to Like Yourself Again.*

She has been interviewed on multiple radio shows about the topic of squirting, including rapper Eminem's Sirius XM channel Shade 45 (All Out Show), as well as on Raw Sex Radio, Erotic Talk Radio, Girl's Eye View, and PPRN.

R. Leigh writes books which share her most intimate experiences in order to help other people learn to accept they are worthy of love, pleasure, and happiness. Her focus is on encouraging others to live a holistic lifestyle, taking into account that mental health, physical health, and other factors affect all aspects of our lives.

Through her writing she hopes to help people all over the world.

Visit her website, www.AuthorRLeigh.com. Follow her

on Facebook, www.facebook.com/AuthorRLeigh and Twitter, @AuthorRLeigh